SIRTFOOD DIET:

Discover how to activate your "skinny gene" with more than 40 Recipes

Table of contents

Chapter I

Introduction

Introduction With the expanding field of exercise physiology or sports medicine, apart from achieving physical fitness and enhanced levels of performance by athletes, physiologists have applied the benefits of exercise in prevention and management of various lifestyle modifiable disease conditions. However, we often overlook the backbone-link between "exercise" and "health". Proper diet and nutrition is the fundamental key to a healthy and positive life. Recent researches have defined nutrition science as "the study of food systems, foods and drinks, and their nutrients and other constituents; and of their interactions within and between all relevant biological, social and environmental systems".

1. With growing awareness among the general public about nutrition and balanced diet, there has been a tremendous change in food pattern, a shift from "junk" food to healthy, less calorie, "zero trans-fat" foods. Even young children are getting motivated to avoid the fast-food chains and switching to foods that would keep them in "picture-perfect figures". But little do they understand that the "zero-trans-fat" foods are not actually fat-free and the authenticity of the advertisements on "nutritious foods" shown on television. Along with awareness of exercise and physical activity, there should be an increase in awareness regarding the aspects of proper nutrition. Childhood and adolescence are the prime areas concerns of nutrition science as they are at the developmental peak years and also formative years for good dietary habits along with exercise and positive outlook in life.

2. Also they lay the basic foundation for future health risks such as hypertension, diabetes mellitus, cancer and other life-style-associated diseases. They are of the concept that "healthy" foods need time to be prepared and that might be the reason why they switch to easily available fast foods. Another common issue is that the healthier foods are priced higher than the less healthy or junk food.

3. However, children should be encouraged to prepare a healthy snack by themselves which would give them motivation and change the notion that it is a time-taking procedure. In the process of preparing their own meal, they could be encouraged to calculate the number of calories contained in the snack and compare it with similar meal when purchased from fast food centers. Not just the younger generation, but also the adults and geriatric population need counseling regarding balanced diet and modifying their diet according to the prevailing disease conditions such as diabetes, hypertension, renal dysfunction, dyslipidemia, obesity, etc.

4. The older population especially needs a lot of attention and care in terms of nutrients to protect them from malnutrition, constipation, and common syndromes of hypertension, diabetes, cancer, renal dysfunction, anemia, osteoporosis, etc.

Thus there is a great need to establish nutrition as a separate branch in physiology, to educate and provide adequate information regarding nutrients and diet at all the stages of life such as infancy, children, adolescents, adults, pregnancy, during lactation and old age. Physiologists are more aware of the body changes, requirements and demands at these different stages so they would be the best guides as nutritionists with a little more education and knowledge in-depth regarding the foods and nutrients available in each food. They can very well prescribe foods to prevent and cure various life-style diseases. This calls for further discussion on how to make them more competent and efficient for this purpose.

Adequate diet of essential nutrients for healthy people

An adequate and balanced diet contributes to achieve or maintain a good state of health. Generally, a balanced diet contains adequate proportions of carbohydrates, fats, and proteins, along with the recommended daily allowances of all essential minerals, vitamins, and health-promoting substances. While carbohydrates and fat mainly provide energy, protein is a structural component of all body cells. The essential nutrients such as a variety of amino acids, fatty acids, vitamins, and minerals have to be provided within the diet. Vitamins and minerals are involved in a large number of metabolic processes.

Nonessential food components such as dietary fibers and phytochemicals are also important for maintenance of health, and possibly also for reducing the risk of chronic disease. Each food group is a characteristic source of certain nutrients: Cereals and legumes mainly provide carbohydrates and protein, vegetables and fruits provide minerals and vitamins, nuts and seeds supply oil and micronutrients, and animal-derived foods are rich in protein.

People in industrialized countries are confronted with a high range of diet-related diseases such as obesity, diabetes, hypertension, certain cancers and coronary heart disease. To achieve an adequate diet and to avoid over nutrition, people have to reduce the consumption of foods high in fat, salt, and energy and low in essential nutrients and therefore increase the intake of foods rich in complex carbohydrates and dietary fiber. In developing countries where traditional diets are frequently adequate, poverty is the main underlying cause of widespread under nutrition and high mortality. Their nutritional problems have to be solved with substantial efforts and changes in the political, economic, and agricultural processes and priorities at national and international levels.

Sirtfood Diet

What is the Sirtfood diet? If you've ever considered following a weight loss diet, make sure you have all the facts first. Dietitian Emer Delaney takes a look at the Sirtfood diet. By Emer Delaney – Dietitian, What is the Sirtfood diet? Launched originally in 2016, the Sirtfood diet remains a hot topic and involves followers adopting a diet rich in 'sirtfoods'. According to the diet's founders, these special foods work by activating specific proteins in the body called sirtuins. Sirtuins are believed to protect cells in the body from dying when they are under stress and are thought to regulate inflammation, metabolism and the aging process. It's thought that sirtuins influence the body's ability to burn fat and boost metabolism, resulting in a seven pound weight loss a week while maintaining muscle. However, some experts believe this is unlikely to be solely fat loss, but will instead reflect changes in glycogen stores from skeletal muscle and the liver.

What are sirtfoods?

Fasting diets have gained a lot of column inches. Studies shows that by fasting followers can expect to lose about 11 pounds in 6 months and experiencing substantial reduction in disease risk. A reduction in our body's energy stores activates what is known as the 'skinny gene'. Fat storage is switched off and our body stops its normal growth processes and go for survival mode. Fat burning is stimulated and the gene involved in the repairs and rejuvenation of our cells are turned on. However a reduction in energy intake provokes hunger, irritability, fatigue and loss of muscle. Enter sirtfoods, a newly discovered group of foods that are rich in special nutrients that, when we consume them, are able to activate the same skinny genes in our bodies as fasting. These genes are known as sirtuins. Sirtfoods are capable of triggering a profoundly beneficial effect in the body, and bit by bit, research has uncovered a collection of these powerful foods.

So what are these magical 'sirtfoods'?
The ten most common include:
1. Green tea
2. Dark chocolate (that is at least 85 per cent cocoa)
3. Apples
4. Citrus fruits
5. Parsley
6. Turmeric
7. Kale
8. Blueberries
9. Capers
10. Red wine

How do Sirtfoods regulate our Metabolism?

Research now shows the benefits of sirtfoods extend further than simply mimicking the effects of caloric restriction. Sirtfoods can have effects on fat burning while simultaneously increasing muscle and enhancing cellular fitness. So far pharmaceutical industries have tried to reduce the benefits of these complex plant nutrients into a single islolated 'drug'. However it likely makes far more sense to eat diets sufficiently rich in these nutrients in their natural food form to reap these exciting benefits.

The science of sirtuins:

They first came to light in a landmark study in 2003 when researchers gave resveratrol, a compound in red grape skin and red wine, to yeast and found it produced the same benefits as caloric restriction without needing to reduce energy intake. Since then researchers have found out that other compounds in red wine exert the same effect, which is now believed to explain the health benefits of red wine consumption and even why people who drink red wine gain less weight.

Each of us possesses an ancient family of genes called sirtuins. Sirtuins are master metabolic regulators that control our ability to burn fat and stay healthy. Sirtuins act as energy sensors within our cells, and get activated when a shortage of energy is detected. Caloric restriction, fasting and exercise all activate our sirtuins genes, but can be hard to stick to and even have drawbacks. By eating a diet rich in sirtfoods you can mimic the effects of fasting and exercise, and achieve the body you want.

Sirtuins and fat burning:

Sirtuins have the power to determine whether we stay lean or get fat. Activating sirt1 inhibits PPAR, blocking the production and storage of fat. Activating sirt1 also promotes PGC-1 alpha which makes more energy factories in our cells and increase fat burning. It also gets our fat cells that specialize in energy storage to behave differently and start disposing of energy.

Sirtuins and muscle building:
By stressing the body, i.e., through fasting, we get increase in free radicals and inflammation. This activity causes the breakdown of our muscle, which we then use for fuel. However, our body does have a system to counter this muscle breakdown; the sirtuins.Sirt1 is a potent inhibitor of muscle breakdown. It keeps free radical and inflammatory chemicals in check leaving our muscles intact and allowing us to continue burning fat instead of muscle for fuel

Fat loss v/s Muscle loss
One pound of muscle weighs exactly like one pound of fat. Yet they look entirely different. One pound of muscle is harder and denser than a pound of body fat. If you gain 6 pounds of muscle and drop six pounds of body fat, your scale weight will be absolutely the same. But you'll definitely be dumbfounded by how much your body changed.

Muscle loss often happens if you focus solely on calorie decrease. Of course, reducing your calorie intake is a basic requirement for weight loss, but it shouldn't be your only goal, or you risk losing your muscle mass. If you're fixing your attention on your diet or upping your cardio in order to burn fat, that focus probably comes at the expense of strength training. It this case, you're most likely to lose tissue weight. That's because calorie restriction often implies macronutrient restriction. Without enough protein in your diet, your body can't rebuild the tissue even if you are strength training. Also, the amount of muscles directly impacts your metabolism.

Skinny gene and its activation:

Genetics play an important role in weight gain and obesity, but even if you didn't inherit lean genes, you can behave as if you did by turning genes on and off to your advantage. The trick is to upgrade how your genes talk to your environment – also known as the gene/environment interaction. Contrary to what we thought even a decade ago, only ten percent of your risk of disease, such as obesity, is genetic; 90 percent is due to your environmental factors, much of which are under your control with the way you eat, drink, move, sleep and think. When it comes to getting older, it turns out that weight gain is one of the most powerful determinants of how fast you are aging.

While your body operates with the 90/10 rule in effect, you can work more wisely with the genes that you have. Many of these genes are known as "famine" genes that evolved to help you extract as much energy as possible from the food you eat, so that you could bank fat and survive a famine. That was a good idea thousands of years ago, but now those same genes can make your jeans tight. While 75 genes increase your chance of obesity, below are the five most important ones that may influence your risk of weight gain and how to change their expression with your lifestyle cues.

Even though you're stuck with the genes you have, you have power over how those genes talk to the rest of your body. Apply these strategies to turn on and off genes to help reach and maintain your ideal weight and extend your health span.

1. FTO OR "FATSO" GENE:
Official Name: Fat mass and obesity associated (FTO) gene
The FTO gene is the gene most strongly associated with your body mass index and, consequently, your risk for obesity and diabetes. When you have the variant that turns off the gene, you may experience poor control of leptin, the hormone of satiety. In other words, you're hungry all of the time. FTO behaves like a fat sensor. People with the FTO variant may be more fat sensitive and tend to eat more food, particularly fat-rich foods, in childhood. People who inherit a faulty gene from each parent weigh about seven pounds more and have a 70 percent greater risk of obesity compared with people who inherit the normal gene from each parent.

Your Task: You can turn on the Fatso gene with exercise, sleeping 7 to 8.5 hours every night, and a low-carbohydrate food plan that's high in fiber. People with the FTO variant, even though they are more predisposed to obesity, they respond just as well to dietary and lifestyle interventions according to a meta-analysis of eight randomized trials of 9,500 people.

2. MCR4 OR "OVERSNACKER" GENE
Official Name: Melanocortin 4 receptor (MCR4)
Their Job: People with this gene variant are more likely to snack too much, in the absence of hunger. They are the people who graze most of the day, taking slivers of cake or tortilla chips. The gene modulates one's appetite for fat, specifically in the amygdala.

Your Task: When you have an increased tendency to snack, I recommend three measured meals, four to six hours apart, with nothing in between. Eat slowly. Resist the urge to snack. Consider more boundaries on your food intake, and if that doesn't work, check out a 12-step program for food addiction such as Overeaters Anonymous or Food Addicts in Recovery.

3. ADRB2 OR "TWICE AS HARD" GENE

Official Name: Adrenergic beta-2 surface receptor (ADRB2)
Their Job: The ADRB2 gene is another famine gene. When turned on, the gene may impair the breaking down of fat, leading to slower metabolism. As a result, you bank fat unnecessarily. Variants may increase the risk of obesity three-fold. Other risks include nocturnal asthma and Type 2 diabetes. Overall, people with this variant, like me, have a lifelong difficult relationship to weight and food. When you have this variation, weight loss takes you twice as long as it takes a normal person. While FTO is associated with body weight, ADRB2 is associated with fat distribution.

Your Task: Exercise helps. So does a mindset Shift. When you accept that it will take you twice as long as your friend to lose weight, it can be strangely calming. Focus on eating the right types and amounts of food with steady discipline. External and internal accountability helps: food journal, group detoxes. Keep in mind that the best path forward is slow and steady weight loss, sustained over time. Track body composition and fat distribution over time.

The science of weight loss

Doubtless the diet will appear to work for some people. But scientific proof of any diet's successes is a very different matter. Of course, the ideal study to consider the effectiveness of a diet on weight loss (or any other outcome, such as ageing) would require a sufficiently large sample – representative of the population we are interested in – and random allocation to a treatment or control group. Outcomes would then be monitored over an adequate period of time with strict control over confounding variables, such as other behaviors that may positively or negatively affect the outcomes of interest (smoking, for example, or exercise).

This research would be limited by methods such as self-reporting and recollection, but would go some way to discovering the effectiveness of this diet. Research of this nature, however, does not exist and we should therefore be cautious when interpreting basic science – after all, human cells in a tissue culture dish probably react very differently to the cells in a living person.

Further doubt is cast over this diet when we consider some of the specific claims. Losses of seven pounds in one week are unrealistic and are very unlikely to reflect changes to body fat. For the first three days, dieters consume around 1000 kcal per day – around 40–50% of what most people require. This will result in a rapid loss of glycogen (a stored form of carbohydrate) from skeletal muscle and the liver.

But for every gram of stored glycogen we also store approximately 2.7 grams of water, and water is heavy. So for all the lost glycogen, we also lose accompanying water – and hence weight. Additionally, diets that are too restrictive are very hard to follow and result in increases in appetite-stimulating hormones, such as ghrelin. Weight (glycogen and water) will therefore return to normal if the urge to eat wins out.

In general, application of the scientific method to the study of nutrition is difficult. It is often not possible to carry out placebo-controlled trials with any degree of ecological validity, and the health outcomes that we are often interested in play out over many years, making research design challenging. Furthermore, studies in large populations depend on surprisingly simplistic and naïve data collection methods such as recollection and self-reporting, which produce notoriously unreliable data. Against this background noise, nutrition research has a difficult job.

Sirtfood and eating habits:

The Sirtfood Diet is based on the principle that certain foods activate sirtuin, a protein in the body that is alleged to help regulate metabolism and offer cell protection to slow down the aging process.

Proponents of the diet say that eating sirtuin-rich foods like green tea, kale, blueberries, salmon, and citrus fruits can give your body a steady metabolic boost. This boost allows you to lose weight fast. Such foods are also packed with polyphenols, which are antioxidants that better your skin and heart.

Sirtfood Diet and Exercise

52% of Americans confessing that they find it easier to do their taxes than to understand how to eat healthily, it's vital to introduce a form of eating that becomes a way of life rather than a one-off fad diet. For some of us it may not be that difficult to lose weight or retain a healthy weight, but the Sirtfood diet can help those who are struggling. But what about combining the Sirtfood diet with exercise, is it advisable to avoid exercise completely or introduce it once you have started the diet?

During the first week or two of the diet where your calorie intake is reduced, it would be sensible to stop or reduce exercise while your body adapts to fewer calories. Listen to your body and if you feel fatigued or have less energy than usual, don't work out. Instead ensure that you remain focused on the principles that apply to a healthy lifestyle such as including adequate daily levels of fiber, protein and fruit and vegetables.

The Sirt diet Principles

With an estimated 650 million obese adults globally, it's important to find healthy eating and exercise regimes that are doable, don't deprive you of everything you enjoy, and don't require you to exercise all week. The Sirtfood diet does just that. The idea is that certain foods will active the 'skinny gene' pathways which are usually activated by fasting and exercise. The good news is that certain food and drink, including dark chocolate and red wine, contain chemicals called polyphenols that activate the genes that mimic the effects of exercise and fasting.

Once the diet becomes a way of life

When you do exercise it's important to consume protein ideally an hour after your workout. Protein repairs muscles after exercise, reduces soreness and can aid recovery. There are a variety of recipes which include protein which will be perfect for post-exercise consumption, such as the Sirt chilli con carne or the turmeric chicken and kale salad. If you want something lighter you could try the Sirt blueberry smoothie and add some protein powder for added benefit.

The type of fitness you do will be down to you, but workouts at home will allow you to choose when to exercise, the types of exercises that suit you and are short and convenient. The Sirtfood diet is great way to change your eating habits, lose weight and feel healthier. The initial few weeks may challenge you but it's important to check which foods are best to eat and which delicious recipes suit you. Be kind to yourself in the first few weeks while your body adapts and take exercise easy if you choose to do it at all. If you are already someone who does moderate or intense exercise then it may be that you can carry on as normal, or manage your fitness in accordance with the change in diet. As with any diet and exercise changes, it's all about the individual and how far you can push yourself.

Chapter 2

Phases of Sirtfood Diet

The diet is divided into two phases;

Phase 1

The initial phase lasts one week and involves restricting calories to 1000kcal for three days, consuming three Sirtfood green juices and one meal rich in sirtfoods each day. The juices include kale, celery, rocket, parsley, green tea and lemon. Meals include turkey escalope with sage, capers and parsley, chicken and kale curry and prawn stir-fry with buckwheat noodles. From day four to seven, energy intakes are increased to 1500kcal comprising of two Sirtfood green juices and two Sirtfood-rich meals a day.

Although the diet promotes healthy foods, it's restrictive in both your food choices and daily Calories, especially during the initial stages. It also involves drinking juice, with the amounts suggested during phase one exceeding the current daily guidelines.

Phase 2

The second phase is known as the maintenance phase which lasts 14 days where steady weight loss occurs. The authors believe it's a sustainable and realistic way to lose weight. However, focusing on weight loss is not what the diet is all about – it's designed to be about eating the best foods nature has to offer. Long term they recommend eating three balanced Sirtfood rich meals a day along with one Sirtfood green juice.

In terms of weight loss and boosting metabolism, people may have experienced a seven pound weight loss on the scales, but in experience this will be fluid. Burning and losing fat takes time so it is extremely unlikely this weight loss is a loss of fat. I would be very cautious of any diet that recommends fast and sudden weight loss as this simply isn't achievable and will more than likely be a loss of fluid. As soon as people return to their regular eating habits, they will regain the weight. Slow and steady weight loss is the key and for this we need to restrict calories and increase our activity levels. Eating balanced regular meals made up of low GI foods, lean protein, fruit and vegetables and keeping well hydrated is the safest way to lose weight.'

Please note: if you're considering attempting any form of diet, please consult your GP first to ensure you can do so without risk to health.

Is the Sirtfood diet good for you?
A pair of authors and health consultants called Aidan Goggins and Glen Matten, whose focus has always been on healthy eating rather than weight loss. In their new book The Sirtfood Diet, the pair lay out a meal plan which involves drinking three Sirtfood green juices a day accompanied by balanced Sirtfood-rich meals, such as a buckwheat and prawn stir-fry or smoked salmon Sirt super salad. Rob says one positive of the diet is that all of the foods you can eat on the plan are good for you, meaning your overall vitamin, mineral and nutrient intake will likely be high.

Benefits of Sirt food diet
1. Better Control of Blood Sugar Levels
2. Decrease Risk of Chronic Disease
3. Anti – Aging Retain

4. Muscle Mass
5. Lose Up to Half a Stone in 7 Days
6. Improvement in Memory Function

Who shouldn't try the Sirtfood diet?
We wouldn't recommend anyone with diabetes try the diet. Plus, it may be hard going if you're highly active. If you do go ahead, he warns to expect side effects like headaches or light-headedness in the first stage of this plan as your body adapts to the lower calorie intake.

Sample Menu:
Phase 1
(Day 1 to 3)
Monday: Sirtfood Green juice+ Sirtfood Green juice+ Sirtfood Green juice+ Buckwheat, Matcha, Rocket and parsley salmon
Tuesday: Sirtfood Green juice+ Sirtfood Green juice+ Sirtfood Green juice+ Parsley walnut and pesto steak
Wednesday: Sirtfood Green juice+ Sirtfood Green juice+ Sirtfood Green juice+ Turkey escalope

(Day 4 to 7)
Thursday: Sirtfood Green juice+ Indian turmeric scramble+ Sirtfood Green juice+ Chicken walnut and parsley pesto
Friday: Sirtfood Green juice+ Sirt smoked salmon+ Sirtfood Green juice+ Strawberry buckwheat Tabbouleh
Saturday: Sirtfood Green juice+ Turmeric chili and kale frittata+ Sirtfood Green juice+ Bun less burger
Sunday: Sirtfood Green juice+ Buckwheat muesli+ Sirtfood Green juice+ Chicken, kale and buck wheat stew

Phase 2

Monday: Sirtfood Green juice+ Sirt greens, chili and turmeric scrambled eggs+ turmeric pancakes+ strawberry buckwheat tabbouleh

Tuesday: Sirtfood Green juice+ Strawberry, Buckwheat and coconut chia bowl+ pulled beef chili with kale, Roasted red onion and buckwheat+ chicken walnut satay, Buckwheat noodles and sirt green

Wednesday: Sirtfood Green juice+ kale, lovage and red onion frittata+ pulled pork salad and sirt avocado mash+ Macha turkey with sirt Aji verde

Thursday: Sirtfood Green juice+ lemon and poppy seed buckwheat waffle+ Indian spiced chicken with sirt green+ Turmeric cauliflower couscous with Moroccan salmon

Friday: Sirtfood Green juice+ sirt shakshuka frittata+ Matcha, lemon and parsley turkey with walnut and kale hummus+ roast lemon and lovage chicken

Saturday: Sirtfood Green juice+ Walnut and strawberry porridge+ Spiced beef brisket with raw sirt slaw+ Buckwheat, turmeric and lemon coated pork

Sunday: Sirtfood Green juice+ turmeric chili and kale frittata+ chicken, kale and buckwheat stew+ sirt smoked salmon+ Buckwheat muesli

Shopping List:
1. Dark Chocolate

A great source of flavonoids, dark chocolate (the kind that's at least 70% cocoa and unprocessed), can improve your health in a number of ways. A small piece of dark chocolate is a great cure for your sugar cravings and it boosts your endorphins and serotonin levels at the same time. The chemicals found in chocolate can also help fight stroke, heart disease, and high blood pressure.

2. Red Wine

Red wine has antioxidants, anti-inflammatory properties and even cancer-fighting potential. Made from purple grape skins and seeds, this beverage is high in polyphenols and resveratrol, which can help protect blood vessels from damage, reduce bad cholesterol, and prevent blood clots. Stick to one glass a day to reap the benefits.

3. Onions

Red onions are not only a low-calorie, flavor-boosting addition to any meal, they may also reduce your risk of developing certain cancers, due to the compound quercetin. Onions are a significant source of antioxidants, and are rich in vitamin C which gives your immune system a welcomed boost.

4. Green Tea

Green tea is made up of antioxidants that help protect our cells from damage and catechins which may play a role in increasing our metabolic rates. Look for matcha green tea since it is made up of crushed tea leaves themselves so it packs a more powerful punch.

5. Blueberries

Blueberries have been found to help lower bad cholesterol, fight signs of aging, reduce inflammation in the body, and help you burn fat. Thanks to the high antioxidant count as well as all the phytonutrients, this dark berry is a snack you can enjoy daily.

6. Coffee

Now you have all the more reason to enjoy your morning cup of coffee. Along with giving you an energy boost, it can also increase your endurance when exercising, reduce your risk of certain diseases, and potentially improve brain function.

7. Parsley

Very high in chlorophyll -- which is a strong antioxidant -- parsley also has alpha-linolenic acid, which is an omega-3 that can fight heart disease and arthritis. The luteolin in this herb may also protect your eyes as well.

8. Turmeric

Another super food, turmeric is often used in ayurvedic treatments, thanks to it being antiseptic, anti-inflammatory, and rich in antioxidants. Curcumin, the compound found in turmeric, not only gives the spice its beautiful bright color, but may also prevent Alzheimer's, certain cancers, and blood clots.

9. Olive Oil

Another ingredient that can lower bad cholesterol, olive oil is full of monounsaturated fatty acids which can also help regulate insulin and blood sugar too. Stick to two tablespoons a day to get the antioxidants your body needs without overdoing it on the calorie front.

Chapter III SIRTFOOD RECIPES

BREAKFAST

1. Aromatic chicken breast with kale and red onions and a tomato and chili salsa

Ingredients:
1. 1⁄4 pound (120g) skinless, boneless chicken breast
2. 2 teaspoons ground turmeric
3. juice of 1⁄4 lemon
4. 1 tablespoon extra virgin olive oil
5. 3⁄4 cup (50g) kale, chopped
6. 1⁄8 cup (20g) red onion, sliced
7. 1 teaspoon chopped fresh ginger
8. 1⁄3 cup (50g) buckwheat

For the salsa:
1. 1 medium tomato (130g)
2. 1 Thai chili, finely chopped
3. 1 tablespoon capers, finely chopped
4. 2 tablespoons (5g) parsley, finely chopped
5. juice of 1⁄4 lemon

Method:
1. To make the salsa, remove the eye from the tomato and chop it very finely, taking care to keep as much of the liquid as possible. Mix with the chili, capers, parsley, and lemon juice. You could put everything in a blender, but the end result is a little different.
2. Heat the oven to 425°F (220°C). Marinate the chicken breast in 1 teaspoon of the turmeric, the lemon juice, and a little oil. Leave for 5 to 10 minutes.
3. Heat an ovenproof frying pan until hot, then add the marinated chicken and cook for a minute or so on each side, until pale golden, then transfer to the oven (place on a baking tray if your pan isn't ovenproof) for 8 to 10 minutes or until cooked through.
4. Remove from the oven, cover with foil, and leave to rest for 5 minutes before serving.
5. Meanwhile, cook the kale in a steamer for 5 minutes. Fry the red onions and the ginger in a little oil, until soft

but not browned, then add the cooked kale and fry for another minute.

6. Cook the buckwheat according to the package instructions with the remaining teaspoon of turmeric. Serve alongside the chicken, vegetables, and salsa.

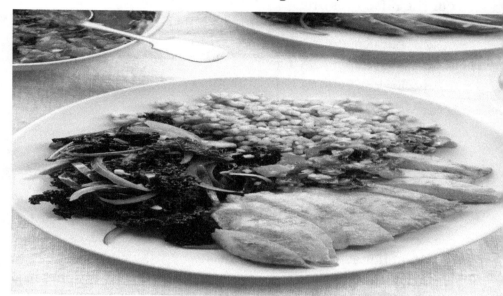

Nutrition Facts: Calories: 226, Carbohydrates: 13.6g, Fat: 8g, Sodium: 351mg, Protein: 27g, Fiber: 4g

2. Buckwheat noodles with chicken kale & miso dressing-Sirtfood

Ingredients:
For the noodles:

1. 2-3 handfuls of kale leaves (removed from the stem and roughly cut)
2. 150 g / 5 oz buckwheat noodles (100% buckwheat, no wheat)
3. 3-4 shiitake mushrooms, sliced
4. 1 teaspoon coconut oil or ghee
5. 1 brown onion, finely diced
6. 1 medium free-range chicken breast, sliced or diced

7. 1 long red chilli, thinly sliced (seeds in or out depending on how hot you like it)
8. 2 large garlic cloves, finely diced
9. 2-3 tablespoons Tamari sauce (gluten-free soy sauce)

For the miso dressing:
1. 1½ tablespoon fresh organic miso
2. 1 tablespoon Tamari sauce
3. 1 tablespoon extra-virgin olive oil
4. 1 tablespoon each of lime juice & sesame oil (optional)

Method:
1. Bring a medium saucepan of water to boil. Add the kale and cook for 1 minute, until slightly wilted. Remove and set aside but reserve the water and bring it back to the boil. Add the soba noodles and cook according to the package instructions (usually about 5 minutes). Rinse under cold water and set aside.
2. In the meantime, pan fry the shiitake mushrooms in a little ghee or coconut oil (about a teaspoon) for 2-3 minutes, until lightly browned on each side. Sprinkle with sea salt and set aside.
3. In the same frying pan, heat more coconut oil or ghee over medium-high heat. Sauté onion and chilli for 2-3 minutes and then add the chicken pieces. Cook 5 minutes over medium heat, stirring a couple of times, then add the garlic, tamari sauce and a little splash of water. Cook for a further 2-3 minutes, stirring frequently until chicken is cooked through.
4. Finally, add the kale and soba noodles and toss through the chicken to warm up.
5. Mix the miso dressing and drizzle over the noodles right at the end of cooking, this way you will keep all those beneficial probiotics in the miso alive and active.

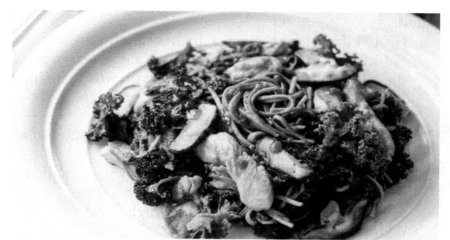

Nutrition Facts: Calories: 105, Carbohydrates: 10.9g, Fat: 5.3g, Sodium: 699mg, Protein: 4.6g, Fiber: 2.1g

3. Asian king prawn stir-fry with buckwheat noodles

Ingredients:

1. 150g shelled raw king prawns, deveined
2. 2 teaspoon tamari
3. 2 teaspoon extra virgin olive oil
4. 75g soba (buckwheat noodles)
5. 1 garlic clove, finely chopped
6. 1 bird's eye chilli, finely chopped
7. 1 teaspoon finely chopped fresh ginger
8. 20g red onions, sliced
9. 40g celery, trimmed and sliced
10. 75g green beans, chopped
11. 50g kale, roughly chopped
12. 100ml chicken stock
13. 5g celery leaves

Method:

1. Heat a frying pan over a high heat, then cook the prawns in 1 teaspoon of the tamari and 1 teaspoon of the oil for 2–3 minutes. Transfer the prawns to a plate. Wipe the pan out with kitchen paper, as you're going to use it again.
2. Cook the noodles in boiling water for 5–8 minutes or as directed on the packet.
3. Drain and set aside. Meanwhile, fry the garlic, chilli and ginger, red onion, celery, beans and kale in the remaining oil over a medium–high heat for 2–3 minutes.
4. Add the stock and bring to the boil, then simmer for a minute or two, until the vegetables are cooked but still crunchy. Add the prawns, noodles and celery leaves to the pan, bring back to the boil then remove from the heat and serve.

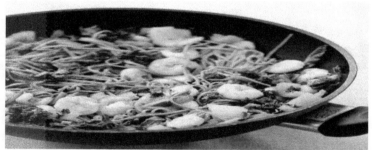

Nutrition Facts: Calories: 423, Carbohydrates: 45.1g, Fat: 17.9g, Sodium: 1.1mg, Protein: 20.7g, Fiber: 0.3g

4. Baked salmon salad with creamy mint dressing

Ingredients:

1. 1 salmon fillet (130g)
2. 40g mixed salad leaves
3. 40g young spinach leaves
4. 2 radishes, trimmed and thinly sliced
5. 5cm piece (50g) cucumber, cut into chunks
6. 2 spring onions, trimmed and sliced

7. 1 small handful (10g) parsley, roughly chopped

For the dressing:
1. 1 teaspoon low-fat mayonnaise
2. 1 tablespoon natural yogurt
3. 1 tablespoon rice vinegar
4. 2 leaves mint, finely chopped
5. Salt and freshly ground black pepper

Method:
1. Preheat the oven to 200°C (180°C fan/Gas 6).
2. Place the salmon fillet on a baking tray and bake for 16–18 minutes until just cooked through. Remove from the oven and set aside. The salmon is equally nice hot or cold in the salad. If your salmon has skin, simply cook skin side down and remove the salmon from the skin using a fish slice after cooking. It should slide off easily when cooked.
3. In a small bowl, mix together the mayonnaise, yogurt, rice wine vinegar, mint leaves and salt and pepper together and leave to stand for at least 5 minutes to allow the flavors to develop.
4. Arrange the salad leaves and spinach on a serving plate and top with the radishes, cucumber, spring onions and parsley. Flake the cooked salmon onto the salad and drizzle the dressing over.

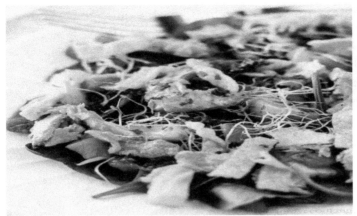

Nutrition Facts: Calories: 250, Carbohydrates: 9g, Fat: 9g, Sodium: 195mg, Protein: 32g,
Fiber: 4g

5. Fragrant Asian hotpot
Ingredients:
1. 1 teaspoon tomato puree
2. 1 star anise, crushed (or 1/4 teaspoon ground anise)
3. Small handful (10g) parsley, stalks finely chopped
4. Small handful (10g) coriander, stalks finely chopped
5. Juice of 1/2 lime
6. 500ml chicken stock, fresh or made with 1 cube
7. 1/2 carrot, peeled and cut into matchsticks
8. 50g broccoli, cut into small florets
9. 50g beansprouts
10. 100g raw tiger prawns
11. 100g firm tofu, chopped
12. 50g rice noodles, cooked according to packet instructions
13. 50g cooked water chestnuts, drained
14. 20g sushi ginger, chopped
15. 1 tablespoon good-quality miso paste

Method:
1. Place the tomato puree, star anise, parsley stalks, coriander stalks, lime juice and chicken stock in a large pan and bring to a simmer for 10 minutes.
2. Add the carrot, broccoli, prawns, tofu, noodles and water chestnuts and simmer gently until the prawns are cooked through.
3. Remove from the heat and stir in the sushi ginger and miso paste. Serve sprinkled with the parsley and coriander leaves.

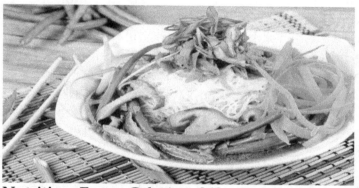

Nutrition Facts: Calories: 262, Carbohydrates: 21g, Fat: 6g, Sodium: 427mg, Protein: 24g, Fiber: 4g

6. Lamb, butternut squash and date tagine

Incredible warming Moroccan spices make this healthy tagine perfect for chilly autumn and winter evenings. Serve with buckwheat for an extra health kick!

Ingredients:
1. 2 tablespoons olive oil
2. 1 red onion, sliced
3. 2cm ginger, grated
4. 3 garlic cloves, grated or crushed
5. 1 teaspoon chilli flakes (or to taste)
6. 2 teaspoons cumin seeds
7. 1 cinnamon stick
8. 2 teaspoons ground turmeric

9. 800g lamb neck fillet, cut into 2cm chunks
10. ½ teaspoon salt
11. 100g medjool dates, pitted and chopped
12. 400g tin chopped tomatoes, plus half a can of water
13. 500g butternut squash, chopped into 1cm cubes
14. 400g tin chickpeas, drained
15. 2 tablespoons fresh coriander (plus extra for garnish)
16. Buckwheat, couscous, flatbreads or rice to serve

Method:
1. Preheat your oven to 140C. Drizzle about 2 tablespoons of olive oil into a large ovenproof saucepan or cast iron casserole dish. Add the sliced onion and cook on a gentle heat, with the lid on, for about 5 minutes, until the onions are softened but not brown.
2. Add the grated garlic and ginger, chilli, cumin, cinnamon and turmeric. Stir well and cook for 1 more minute with the lid off. Add a splash of water if it gets too dry.
3. Next add in the lamb chunks. Stir well to coat the meat in the onions and spices and then add the salt, chopped dates and tomatoes, plus about half a can of water (100-200ml).
4. Bring the tagine to the boil and then put the lid on and put in your preheated oven for 1 hour and 15 minutes.
5. Thirty minutes before the end of the cooking time, add in the chopped butternut squash and drained chickpeas. Stir everything together, put the lid back on and return to the oven for the final 30 minutes of cooking.
6. When the tagine is ready, remove from the oven and stir through the chopped coriander. Serve with buckwheat, couscous, flatbreads or basmati rice.

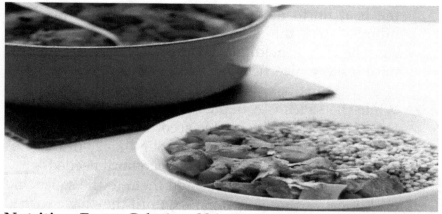

Nutrition Facts: Calories: 226, Carbohydrates: 13.6g, Fat: 8g, Sodium: 351mg, Protein: 27g, Fiber: 4g

7. Prawn Arrabbiata

Ingredients:

1. 125-150 g Raw or cooked prawns (Ideally king prawns)
2. 65 g Buckwheat pasta
3. 1 tablespoon Extra virgin olive oil

For arrabbiata sauce:

1. 40 g Red onion, finely chopped
2. 1 Garlic clove, finely chopped
3. 30 g Celery, finely chopped
4. 1 Bird's eye chilli, finely chopped
5. 1 teaspoon Dried mixed herbs
6. 1 teaspoon extra virgin olive oil
7. 2 tablespoon White wine (optional)
8. 400 g Tinned chopped tomatoes
9. 1 tablespoon Chopped parsley

Method:

1. Fry the onion, garlic, celery and chilli and dried herbs in the oil over a medium–low heat for 1–2 minutes. Turn

the heat up to medium, add the wine and cook for 1 minute. Add the tomatoes and leave the sauce to simmer over a medium–low heat for 20–30 minutes, until it has a nice rich consistency. If you feel the sauce is getting too thick simply add a little water.

2. While the sauce is cooking bring a pan of water to the boil and cook the pasta according to the packet instructions. When cooked to your liking, drain, toss with the olive oil and keep in the pan until needed.

3. If you are using raw prawns add them to the sauce and cook for a further 3–4 minutes, until they have turned pink and opaque, add the parsley and serve. If you are using cooked prawns add them with the parsley, bring the sauce to the boil and serve.

4. Add the cooked pasta to the sauce, mix thoroughly but gently and serve.

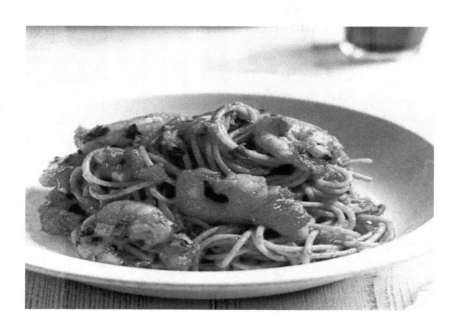

Nutrition Facts: Calories: 415, Carbohydrates: 57g, Fat: 10g, Sodium: 549mg, Protein: 23g, Fiber: 5g

8. Coronation chicken salad

Ingredients:
1. 75 g Natural yoghurt
2. Juice of 1/4 of a lemon
3. 1 teaspoon Coriander, chopped
4. 1 teaspoon Ground turmeric
5. 1/2 teaspoon Mild curry powder
6. 100 g Cooked chicken breast, cut into bite-sized pieces
7. 6 Walnut halves, finely chopped
8. 1 Medjool date, finely chopped
9. 20 g Red onion, diced
10. 1 Bird's eye chilli
11. 40 g Rocket, to serve

Method:
1. Mix the yoghurt, lemon juice, coriander and spices together in a bowl.
2. Add all the remaining ingredients and serve on a bed of the rocket.

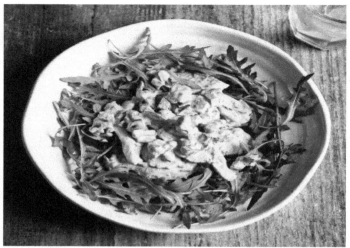

Nutrition Facts: Calories: 362, Carbohydrates: 7.3g, Fat: 24.9g, Sodium: 80mg, Protein: 29.4g, Fiber: 2.6g

9. Turkey Escalope

Ingredients:

1. 1 2 lb turkey breast, on the bone (or same weight of turkey scallopini)
2. salt and pepper
3. ¾ cup all purpose flour
4. 2 eggs
5. ¼ cup cold
6. 1 cup milk
7. 1 teaspoon dry breadcrumbs
8. 1 tablespoon finely chopped fresh thyme
9. 2 tablespoon butter
10. 2 tablespoon olive oil
11. 1 lemon

Method:

1. With a sharp knife, take turkey breast off the bone. Slice turkey against the grain into thin slices. Pound turkey (placed inside a resealable bag with a meat tenderizer until thin but without tearing.

2. To prepare turkey for breading, stir a little salt & pepper into our in a lat bowl. Whisk eggs with milk and season lightly. Season breadcrumbs lightly and mix in thyme in a third at bowl. Preheat a large sauté pan over medium-high heat and melt 1 tablespoon butter and 1 tablespoon oil.

3. Dip first turkey escalope in our, coating both sides. Shake off excess our, then dip into egg mixture, coating well. Shake off excess, then coat completely in breadcrumbs. Add to skillet and repeat with other escalopes to fill pan without crowding. Cook about 4 minutes on each side, until cooked through. Place cooked cutlets on a platter or baking tray and hold in a 325F oven while preparing remaining escalopes. Add remaining butter and oil and cook remaining turkey escalopes. Squeeze lemon juice over immediately before serving.

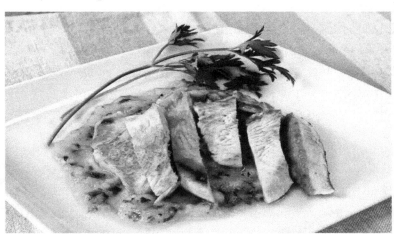

Nutrition Facts: Calories: 139, Carbohydrates: 12.3g, Fat: 7.9g, Sodium: 364mg, Protein: 4.7g, Fiber: 1.2g

10. Baked potatoes with spicy chickpea stew

Kind of Mexican Mole meets North African Tagine, this Spicy Chickpea Stew is unbelievably delicious and makes a great topping for baked potatoes, plus it just happens to be vegetarian, vegan, gluten free and dairy free. And it contains chocolate.

Ingredients:
1. 4-6 baking potatoes, pricked all over
2. 2 tablespoons olive oil
3. 2 red onions, finely chopped
4. 4 cloves garlic, grated or crushed
5. 2cm ginger, grated
6. ½ -2 teaspoons chilli flakes
7. 2 tablespoons cumin seeds
8. 2 tablespoons turmeric
9. Splash of water
10. 2 x 400g tins chopped tomatoes
11. 2 tablespoons unsweetened cocoa powder
12. 2 x 400g tins chickpeas, including the chickpea water
13. 2 yellow peppers, chopped into bite size pieces
14. 2 tablespoons parsley plus extra for garnish
15. Salt and pepper to taste (optional)

Method:
1. Preheat the oven to 200C, meanwhile you can prepare all your ingredients.
2. When the oven is hot enough put your baking potatoes in the oven and cook for 1 hour or until they are done how you like them.

3. Once the potatoes are in the oven, place the olive oil and chopped red onion in a large wide saucepan and cook gently, with the lid on for 5 minutes, until the onions are soft but not brown.

4. Remove the lid and add the garlic, ginger, cumin and chilli. Cook for a further minute on a low heat, then add the turmeric and a very small splash of water and cook for another minute, taking care not to let the pan get too dry.

5. Next, add in the tomatoes, cocoa powder (or cacao), chickpeas (including the chickpea water) and yellow pepper. Bring to the boil, then simmer on a low heat for 45 minutes until the sauce is thick and unctuous (but don't let it burn!). The stew should be done at roughly the same time as the potatoes.

6. Finally stir in the 2 tablespoons of parsley, and some salt and pepper if you wish, and serve the stew on top of the baked potatoes, perhaps with a simple side salad.

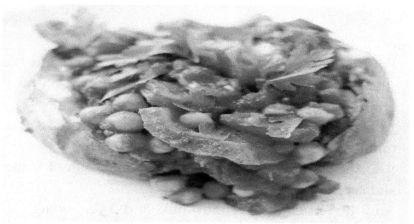

Nutrition Facts: Calories: 314, Carbohydrates: 57g, Fat: 6.4g, Sodium: 658mg, Protein: 9.8g, Fiber: 9.4g

11. Kale and red onion dhal with buckwheat

Delicious and very nutritious this Kale and Red Onion Dhal with Buckwheat is quick and easy to make and naturally gluten free, dairy free, vegetarian and vegan.

Ingredients:
1. 1 tablespoon olive oil
2. 1 small red onion, sliced
3. 3 garlic cloves, grated or crushed
4. 2 cm ginger, grated
5. 1 birds eye chilli, deseeded and finely chopped
6. 2 teaspoons turmeric
7. 2 teaspoons garam masala
8. 160g red lentils
9. 400ml coconut milk
10. 200ml water
11. 100g kale (or spinach would be a great alternative)
12. 160g buckwheat (or brown rice)

Method:
1. Put the olive oil in a large, deep saucepan and add the sliced onion. Cook on a low heat, with the lid on for 5 minutes until softened.
2. Add the garlic, ginger and chilli and cook for 1more minute.
3. Add the turmeric, garam masala and a splash of water and cook for 1 more minute.
4. Add the red lentils, coconut milk, and 200ml water (do this simply by half filling the coconut milk can with water and tipping it into the saucepan).
5. Mix everything together thoroughly and cook for 20 minutes over a gently heat with the lid on. Stir

occasionally and add a little more water if the dhal starts to stick.

6. After 20 minutes add the kale, stir thoroughly and replace the lid, cook for a further 5 minutes (1-2 minutes if you use spinach instead!)

7. About 15 minutes before the curry is ready, place the buckwheat in a medium saucepan and add plenty of boiling water. Bring the water back to the boil and cook for 10 minutes (or a little longer if you prefer your buckwheat softer. Drain the buckwheat in a sieve and serve with the dhal.

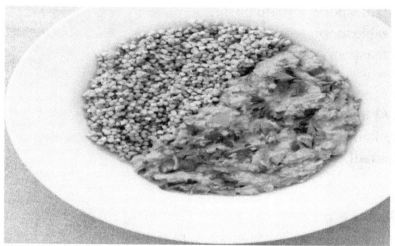

Nutrition Facts: Calories: 402, Carbohydrates: 71g, Fat: 7g, Sodium: 43mg, Protein: 18g, Fiber: 18g

12. Bunless burger recipe
Ingredients:
For the burgers:
1. 1 lb ground beef
2. 1 tablespoon ghee salt and pepper

For the toppings and "bun":
1. 1 onion, sliced into rings
2. 1 tablespoon ghee
3. 1 tomato, sliced
4. 1 dill pickle, sliced into rounds
5. 1 head iceberg lettuce

For the sauce:
1. 2 tablespoon tomato paste
2. 1 tablespoon white vinegar
3. 1 teaspoon mustard
4. 1 teaspoon coconut aminos
5. 1/4 teaspoon garlic powder
6. 1/4 teaspoon onion powder
7. 1/4 cup mayo
8. 1 small dill pickle, finely diced

Method:
1. Start by making the sauce. Combine all of the sauce ingredients in a bowl and mix well with a whisk. Refrigerate while you make the burgers.
2. Form beef into burger patties. You want very thin patties, about 1/4 inch thick. 1 lb of beef will make about 4 of these patties. They will be very large and thin (but will shrink a lot when cooking). Season the patties with salt and pepper on both sides and set aside.
3. Slice onion as noted and heat a medium skillet over medium-low heat and add 1 tablespoon of ghee. Add the onion to cook, stirring occasionally, until browned and caramelized. This should take about 15 minutes

and be finished about the same time as the burgers. If they cook to fast or finish early, just simmer on low until the burgers are ready.

4. Prep the toppings for the burgers as noted. For the buns, cut the iceberg lettuce head into fourths. Cut off the bottom "stem" of each wedge of lettuce. Remove the thick inner pieces, leaving the outer leaves. You'll split these leaves to form your top and bottom "bun".

5. Cook over medium-high heat on a grill or heat a large skillet over medium-high heat and add 1 tablespoon ghee. Once the ghee is hot and shimmering (or the grill is hot), add the burgers to cook for 3-4 minutes per side, or until cooked to your liking. If using a skillet, you may have to cook burgers in batches, two at a time.

6. Now, assemble your burgers. Put 1/2 of the lettuce wedge on a plate and add a tomato slice and some pickles at the bottom. Top with a burger patty and spread some sauce over the top. Add on some onions and top with more sauce if desired. Top with the other 1/2 of the lettuce wedge to form a burger. Pick it up with both hands and enjoy!

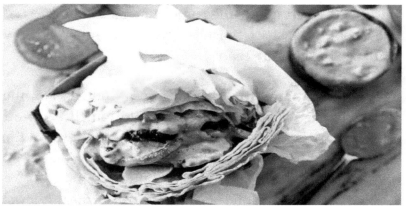

Nutrition Facts: Calories: 154, Carbohydrates: 25.3g, Fat: 1.6g, Sodium: 195mg, Protein: 9.1g, Fiber: 5.1g

13. Mushroom Scramble Egg
Ingredients:
1. 2 eggs
2. 1 teaspoon ground turmeric
3. 1 teaspoon mild curry powder
4. 20g kale, roughly chopped
5. 1 teaspoon extra virgin olive oil
6. ½ bird's eye chilli, thinly sliced
7. handful of button mushrooms, thinly sliced
8. 5g parsley, finely chopped

Method:
1. Mix the turmeric and curry powder and add a little water until you have achieved a light paste.
2. Steam the kale for 2– 3 minutes. Heat the oil in a frying pan over a medium heat and fry the chilli and mushrooms for 2– 3 minutes until they have started to brown and soften.

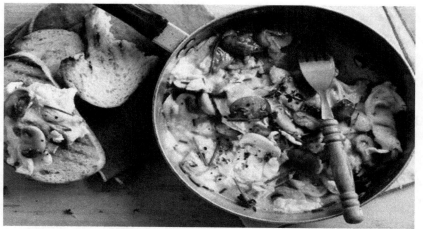

Nutrition Facts: Calories: 140, Carbohydrates: 1.4g, Fat: 9.6g, Sodium: 0mg, Protein: 12g, Fiber: 0g

14. Chargrilled beef with a red wine jus, onion rings, garlic kale and herb roasted potatoes

Ingredients:

1. 100g potatoes, peeled and cut into 2cm dice
2. 1 tablespoon extra virgin olive oil
3. 5g parsley, finely chopped
4. 50g red onion, sliced into rings
5. 50g kale, sliced
6. 1 garlic clove, finely chopped
7. 150g x 3.5cm-thick beef fillet steak or 2cm-thick sirloin steak
8. 40ml red wine
9. 150ml beef stock
10. 1 teaspoon tomato puree
11. 1 teaspoon corn flour, dissolved in 1 tablespoon water

Method:

1. Heat the oven to 220°C/gas 7. Place the potatoes in a saucepan of boiling water, bring back to the boil and cook for 4–5 minutes, then drain.

2. Place in a roasting tin with 1 teaspoon of the oil and roast in the hot oven for 35–45 minutes. Turn the potatoes every 10 minutes to ensure even cooking. When cooked, remove from the oven, sprinkle with the chopped parsley and mix well.

3. Fry the onion in 1 teaspoon of the oil over a medium heat for 5–7 minutes, until soft and nicely caramelized. Keep warm.

4. Steam the kale for 2–3 minutes then drain.

5. Fry the garlic gently in ½ teaspoon of oil for 1 minute, until soft but not colored. Add the kale and fry for a further 1–2 minutes, until tender. Keep warm.

6. Heat an ovenproof frying pan over a high heat until smoking. Coat the meat in ½ a teaspoon of the oil and fry in the hot pan over a medium–high heat according to how you like your meat done. If you like your meat medium it would be better to sear the meat and then transfer the pan to an oven set at 220°C/gas 7 and finish the cooking that way for the prescribed times. Remove the meat from the pan and set aside to rest.

7. Add the wine to the hot pan to bring up any meat residue. Bubble to reduce the wine by half, until syrupy and with a concentrated flavor.

8. Add the stock and tomato purée to the steak pan and bring to the boil, then add the corn flour paste to thicken your sauce, adding it a little at a time until you have your desired consistency. Stir in any of the juices from the rested steak and serve with the roasted potatoes, kale, onion rings and red wine sauce.

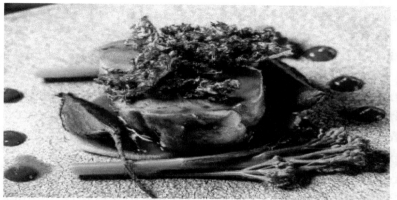

Nutrition Facts: Calories: 207, Carbohydrates: 7.8g, Fat: 10.8g, Sodium: 0mg, Protein: 19.7g, Fiber: 0g

15. Kale, edamame and tofu curry

A warming and wintry curry. Easy to keep either refrigerated or frozen for another day.

Ingredients:

1. 1 tablespoon rapeseed oil
2. 1 large onion, chopped
3. 4 cloves garlic, peeled and grated
4. 1 large thumb (7cm) fresh ginger, peeled and grated
5. 1 red chilli, deseeded and thinly sliced
6. 1/2 teaspoon ground turmeric
7. 1/4 teaspoon cayenne pepper
8. 1 teaspoon paprika
9. 1/2 teaspoon ground cumin
10. 1 teaspoon salt
11. 250g dried red lentils
12. 1 liter boiling water
13. 50g frozen soya edamame beans
14. 200g firm tofu, chopped into cubes
15. 2 tomatoes, roughly chopped
16. Juice of 1 lime

17. 200g kale leaves, stalks removed and torn

Method:
1. Put the oil in a heavy-bottomed pan over a low-medium heat. Add the onion and cook for 5 minutes before adding the garlic, ginger and chilli and cooking for a further 2 minutes. Add the turmeric, cayenne, paprika, cumin and salt. Stir through before adding the red lentils and stirring again.
2. Pour in the boiling water and bring to a hearty simmer for 10 minutes, then reduce the heat and cook for a further 20-30 minutes until the curry has a thick '•porridge' consistency.
3. Add the soya beans, tofu and tomatoes and cook for a further 5 minutes. Add the lime juice and kale leaves and cook until the kale is just tender.

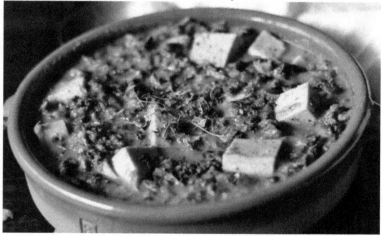

Nutrition Facts: Calories: 157, Carbohydrates: 14.2g, Fat: 7.1g, Sodium: 22.9mg, Protein: 13g, Fiber: 3.1g

16. Buckwheat pasta salad

Ingredients:

1. 50g buckwheat pasta(cooked according to the packet instructions)
2. large handful of rocket
3. small handful of basil leaves
4. 8 cherry tomatoes, halved
5. 1/2 avocado, diced
6. 10 olives
7. 1 tablespoon extra virgin olive oil
8. 20g pine nuts

Method:

1. Gently combine all the ingredients except the pine nuts and arrange on a plate or in a bowl, then scatter the pine nuts over the top

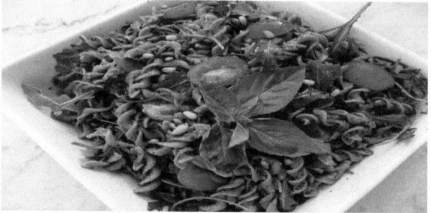

Nutrition Facts: Calories: 113, Carbohydrates: 2g, Fat: 9g, Sodium: 0mg, Protein: 6g, Fiber: 0g

17. Shakshuka recipe

Easy shakshuka made with eggs that are gently poached in a simmering mixture of tomatoes, bell peppers, onions, and garlic. A few warm spices and some fresh herbs complete this satisfying one-skillet dish!

Ingredients:
1. Extra virgin olive oil 1
2. large yellow onion, chopped
3. 2 green peppers, chopped
4. 2 garlic cloves, peeled, chopped
5. 1 teaspoon ground coriander
6. 1 teaspoon sweet paprika
7. 1/2 teaspoon ground cumin
8. Pinch red pepper flakes (optional)
9. Salt and pepper
10. 6 Vine-ripe tomatoes, chopped
11. 1/2 cup tomato sauce
12. 6 large eggs
13. 1/4 cup chopped fresh parsley leaves
14. 1/4 cup chopped fresh mint leaves

Method:
1. Heat 3 tablespoon olive oil in a large cast iron skillet. Add the onions, green peppers, garlic, spices, pinch salt and pepper. Cook, stirring occasionally, until the vegetables have softened, about 5 minutes.
2. Add the tomatoes and tomato sauce. Cover and let simmer for about 15 minutes. Uncover and cook a bit longer to allow the mixture to reduce and thicken. Taste and adjust the seasoning to your liking.

3. Using a wooden spoon, make 6 indentations, or "wells," in the tomato mixture (make sure the indentations are spaced out). Gently crack an egg into each indention.
4. Reduce the heat, cover the skillet, and cook on low until the egg whites are set.
5. Uncover and add the fresh parsley and mint. You can add more black pepper or crushed red pepper, if you like. Serve with warm pita, challah bread, or your choice of crusty bread.

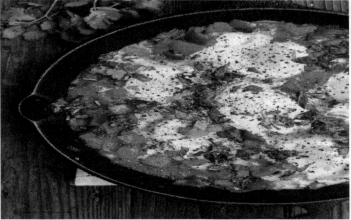

Nutrition Facts: Calories: 256, Carbohydrates: 25.1g, Fat: 14g, Sodium: 446mg, Protein: 4.6g, Fiber: 7.7g

18. Sirt muesli

Ingredients:
1. 20g buckwheat flakes
2. 10g buckwheat puffs
3. 15g coconut flakes or desiccated coconut
4. 40g Medjool dates, pitted and chopped
5. 15g walnuts, chopped
6. 10g cocoa nibs
7. 100g strawberries, hulled and chopped
8. 100g plain Greek yoghurt (or vegan alternative, such as soya or coconut yoghurt)

Method:
1. Mix all of the above ingredients together, only adding the yoghurt and strawberries before serving if you are making it in bulk

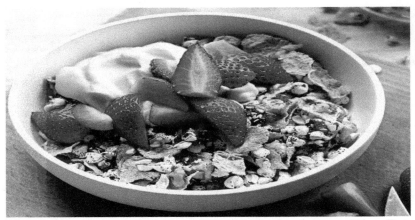

Nutrition Facts: Calories: 515, Carbohydrates: 76g, Fat: 23g, Sodium: 0mg, Protein: 37g, Fiber: 2g

19. Tuscan Bean Stew

Ingredients:
1. 1 tablespoon extra virgin olive oil
2. 50g red onion, finely chopped
3. 30g carrot, peeled and finely chopped
4. 30g celery, trimmed and finely chopped
5. 1 garlic clove, finely chopped
6. ½ bird's eye chilli, finely chopped (optional)
7. 1 teaspoon herbes de Provence
8. 200ml vegetable stock
9. 1 x 400g tin chopped Italian tomatoes
10. 1 teaspoon tomato puree
11. 200g tinned mixed beans
12. 50g kale, roughly chopped
13. 1 tablespoon roughly chopped parsley
14. 40g buckwheat

Method:
1. Place the oil in a medium saucepan over a low-medium heat and gently fry the onion, carrot, celery, garlic, chilli(if using) and herbs, until the onion is soft but not colored.
2. Add the stock, tomatoes and tomato purée and bring to the boil. Add the beans and simmer for 30 minutes. Add the kale and cook for another 5–10 minutes, until tender, then add the parsley.
3. Meanwhile, cook the buckwheat according to the packet instructions, drain and then serve with the stew.

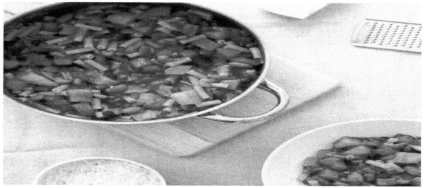

Nutrition Facts: Calories: 264, Carbohydrates: 45.8g, Fat: 2.7g, Sodium: 99mg, Protein: 17.1g, Fiber: 16.8g

20. Salmon Sirt Super Salad

Ingredients:

1. 50g rocket
2. 50g chicory leaves
3. 100g smoked salmon slices (you can also use lentils, cooked chicken breast or tinned tuna)
4. 80g avocado, peeled, stoned and sliced
5. 40g celery, sliced
6. 20g red onion, sliced
7. 15g walnuts, chopped
8. 1 tablespoon capers
9. 1 large Medjool date, pitted and chopped
10. 1 tablespoon extra-virgin olive oil
11. Juice ¼ lemon
12. 10g parsley, chopped
13. 10g celery leaves, chopped

Method:

1. Arrange the salad leaves on a large plate. Mix all the remaining ingredients together and serve on top of the leaves.

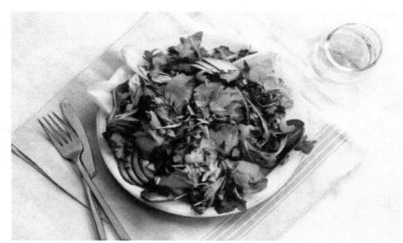

Nutrition Facts: Calories: 250, Carbohydrates: 9g, Fat: 9g, Sodium: 195mg, Protein: 32g, Fiber: 4g

LUNCH

21. Pulled Pork, Cabbage and Arugula Salad

Pulled pork, cabbage and arugula salad with citrus lime vinaigrette is a hearty, flavorful and healthy salad recipe. It's a great way to enjoy pulled pork with lots of veggies!

Ingredients:
1. 4 cups pulled pork
2. 3 cups sliced red cabbage
3. 1 cup baby arugula
4. 1 medium carrot grated
5. 1 small bunch cilantro chopped
6. 1/3 cup sliced almonds
7. 1 Citrus Lime Vinaigrette

Method:
1. Add all of the ingredients to a mixing bowl, drizzle with the Citrus Lime Vinaigrette and stir together.

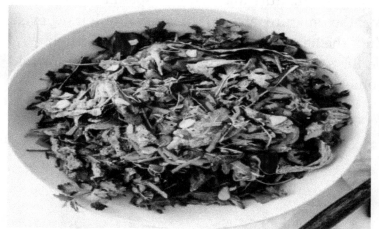

Nutrition Facts: Calories: 345, Carbohydrates: 35g, Fat: 20g, Sodium: 485mg, Protein: 27g, Fiber: 1.8g

22. Smoked Salmon Omelette

Try this quick and easy Sirtfood dish packed with flavor and goodness.

Ingredients:

1. 2 Medium eggs
2. 100 g Smoked salmon, sliced
3. 1/2 teaspoon Capers
4. 10 g Rocket, chopped
5. 1 teaspoon Parsley, chopped
6. 1 teaspoon extra virgin olive oil

Method:

1. Crack the eggs into a bowl and whisk well.
2. Add the salmon, capers, rocket and parsley.
3. Heat the olive oil in a non-stick frying pan until hot but not smoking.
4. Add the egg mixture and, using a spatula or fish slice, move the mixture around the pan until it is even. Reduce the heat and let the omelette cook through.
5. Slide the spatula around the edges and roll up or fold the omelette in half to serve.

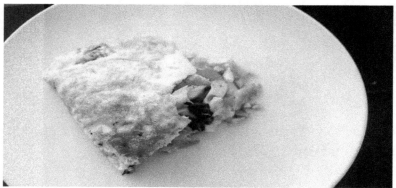

Nutrition Facts: Calories: 117, Carbohydrates: 0g, Fat: 4.3g, Sodium: 784mg, Protein: 18.3g, Fiber: 0g

23. Miso marinated cod with stir fried greens & sesame

Ingredients:
1. 20g miso
2. 1 tablespoon mirin
3. 1 tablespoon extra virgin olive oil
4. 200g skinless cod fillet
5. 20g red onion, sliced
6. 40g celery, sliced
7. 1 garlic clove, finely chopped
8. 1 bird's eye chilli, finely chopped
9. 1 teaspoon finely chopped fresh ginger
10. 60g green beans 50g kale, roughly chopped
11. 1 teaspoon sesame seeds
12. 5g parsley, roughly chopped
13. 1 tablespoon tamari
14. 30g buckwheat
15. 1 teaspoon ground turmeric

Method:
1. Mix the miso, mirin and 1 teaspoon of the oil. Rub all over the cod and leave to marinate for 30 minutes.
2. Heat the oven to 220°C/gas 7. Bake the cod for 10 minutes.
3. Meanwhile, heat a large frying pan or wok with the remaining oil. Add the onion and stir-fry for a few minutes, then add the celery, garlic, chilli, ginger, green beans and kale. Toss and fry until the kale is tender and cooked through. You may need to add a little water to the pan to aid the cooking process.

4. Cook the buckwheat according to the packet instructions with the turmeric for 3 minutes.
5. Add the sesame seeds, parsley and tamari to the stir-fry and serve with the greens and fish.

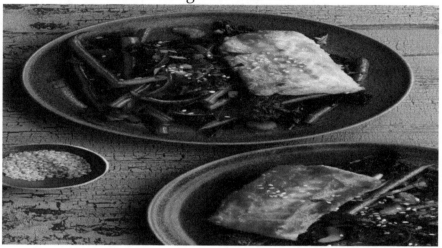

Nutrition Facts: Calories: 250, Carbohydrates: 12g, Fat: 3g, Sodium: 100mg, Protein: 43g, Fiber: 0g

24. Chinese-style pork with pak choi
Ingredients:
1.
   00g firm tofu, cut into large cubes
2.
   tablespoon corn flour
3.
   tablespoon water
4.
   25ml chicken stock
5.
   tablespoon rice wine

6.

    tablespoon tomato puree

7.

    teaspoon brown sugar

8.

    tablespoon soy sauce

9.

    clove garlic, peeled and crushed

10.

    thumb (5cm) fresh ginger, peeled and grated

11.

    tablespoon rapeseed oil

12.

    00g shiitake mushrooms, sliced

13.

    shallot, peeled and sliced

14.

    00g pak choi or choi sum, cut into thin slices

15.

    00g pork mince (10% fat)

16.

    00g beansprouts

17.

    arge handful (20g) parsley, chopped

Method:

1.

    ay out the tofu on kitchen paper, cover with more kitchen paper and set aside.

2.

    n a small bowl, mix together the corn flour and water, removing all lumps. Add the chicken stock, rice wine, tomato puree, brown sugar and soy sauce. Add the crushed garlic and ginger and stir together. In a wok or large frying pan, heat the oil to a high temperature.

3.

dd the shiitake mushrooms and stir-fry for 2–3 minutes until cooked and glossy. Remove the mushrooms from the pan with a slotted spoon and set aside.

4.

dd the tofu to the pan and stir-fry until golden on all sides. Remove with a slotted spoon and set aside.

5.

dd the shallot and pak choi to the wok, stir-fry for 2 minutes, then add the mince. Cook until the mince is cooked through, then add the sauce, reduce the heat a notch and allow the sauce to bubble round the meat for a minute or two.

6.

dd the beansprouts, shiitake mushrooms and tofu to the pan and warm through. Remove from the heat, stir through the parsley and serve immediately.

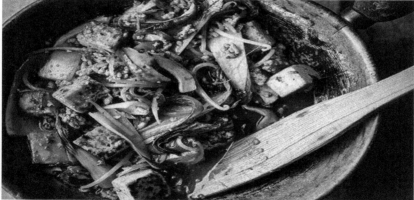

Nutrition Facts: Calories: 323, Carbohydrates: 7.3g, Fat: 21g, Sodium: 1012mg, Protein: 24.1g, Fiber: 1.3g

25. Fish in Red Wine Butter Sauce

A perfect red snapper in a simple but elegant red wine and butter sauce. A delicious combination of wine and fish! Fish tastes better in wine and butter, doesn't it?

Ingredients:

For the fish:

1. 1 Red snapper fillet
2. Salt
3. Pepper
4. Olive oil

For the red wine butter sauce:

1. 1/2 Liter Red wine
2. Few sprigs Thyme
3. 1 Bay leaf
4. A pinch of Sugar
5. 1 teaspoon Mustard sauce
6. 2 tablespoon Butter
7. Thyme, to garnish
8. Reduced balsamic vinegar, to garnish

Method:

1. Marinate the fillet with some salt, pepper and olive oil. Pan fry it in a teaspoon of olive oil for a minute or two on each side.
2. In a heavy bottomed pan add 1/2 liter red wine. Add thyme, bay leaf, sugar and mustard sauce. Let it reduce.
3. Once the sauce starts to reduce add butter and whisk it. Let it simmer.

4. Plating up: Place the pan fried fish fillets on a plate. Pour over some red wine sauce and reduced balsamic vinegar. Garnish with some thyme. Serve.

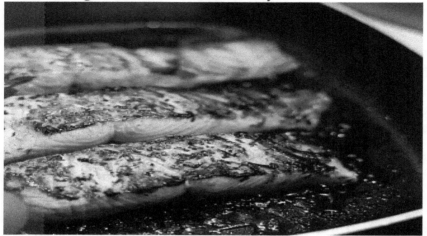

Nutrition Facts: Calories: 107, Carbohydrates: 10.4g, Fat: 0.3g, Sodium: 6.8mg, Protein: 0.5g, Fiber: 2.2g

26. Chicken Cacciatore with Red Wine

This "hunter style" dish is beloved not just in Italy, but all around the world. This hearty recipe has all the bright and sunny flavors of the Italian countryside.

Ingredients:
1. Salt
2. Pepper
3. 4 boneless skinless chicken breasts
4. 1/4 all-purpose flour
5. 3 tablespoons olive oil
6. 2 tablespoons butter
7. 1 medium onion, chopped
8. 1 medium red bell pepper, seeded, chopped
9. 3 cloves garlic, finely chopped
10. 1 cup red wine
11. 1 can (28 oz) crushed tomatoes

12. 1 cup chicken broth (from 32-oz)
13. 1 teaspoon dried oregano leaves
14. 2 tablespoons julienned fresh basil leaves

Method:

1. Sprinkle salt and pepper over chicken breasts; coat chicken with flour. In Dutch oven, heat oil over medium-high heat. Add chicken; cook until browned on both sides. Remove chicken from Dutch oven; place on plate. Set aside.

2. In same Dutch oven, melt butter over medium heat. Add onion, bell pepper and garlic; cook and stir 5 minutes. Add red wine; cook until reduced in half.

3. Stir in tomatoes, broth and oregano. Place chicken over tomatoes. Heat to boiling. Reduce heat to medium-low; simmer about 20 minutes or until juice of chicken is clear when center of thickest part is cut (165°F).

4. Serve chicken over mashed potatoes or spaghetti, spooning sauce over chicken. Sprinkle with basil

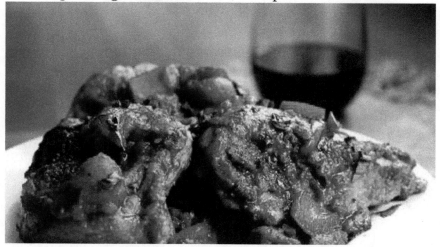

Nutrition Facts: Calories: 290, Carbohydrates: 38.1g, Fat: 4g, Sodium: 150mg, Protein: 25g, Fiber: 5.1g

27. Lemon parsley rice salad

A bright and vibrant dish that pairs well with poultry or seafood, you're going to love this simple lemon and parsley rice salad.

Ingredients:

1. 3 cups cooked rice (1 cup uncooked)
2. 1 tablespoon fresh lemon juice
3. 1 1/2 teaspoons lemon zest
4. 1/4 cup extra virgin olive oil
5. Salt, to taste
6. Freshly ground black pepper, to taste
7. 1 cup tightly packed, finely chopped Italian flat leaf parsley
8. 1/2 small sweet Italian frying pepper or bell pepper, cut into 1/4-inch dice
9. Lemon wedges for serving (optional)

Method:

1. If you have not already, prepare the rice. If it's ready to go, add a splash of water and heat it up in a microwave-safe bowl.
2. To make the dressing, combine the lemon juice and lemon zest in a large wooden salad bowl, and whisk in the olive oil. Add salt and pepper to taste.
3. Add the rice, parsley, and diced pepper. Mix well. Season with additional salt and pepper, to taste.
4. Serve warm or at room temperature with lemon wedges on the side.

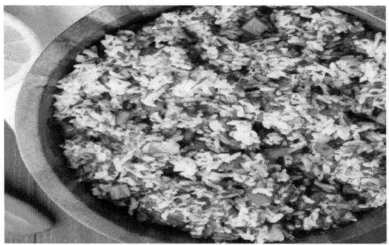

Nutrition Facts: Calories: 387, Carbohydrates: 55g, Fat: 14.9g, Sodium: 15mg, Protein: 9.8g, Fiber: 5.8g

28. Parsley Pesto Pasta

Forget expensive basil pasta, this quick and easy parsley pesto pasta packs a huge flavor punch and costs pennies.

Ingredients:
1. 1 lb. fettuccini
2. 1 bunch Italian parsley
3. 1/2 cup grated parmesan
4. 2 tablespoon lemon juice
5. 2 cloves garlic
6. 1/4 teaspoon salt
7. 1/2 cup olive oil

Method:
1. Rinse the parsley well and shake off as much water as possible. Remove the leaves from the stems and place

them into the food processor. Also add the garlic (peeled), parmesan cheese, and lemon juice. Pulse until there are no large chunks of garlic left.

2. Slowly add the olive oil through the spout on the lid as you continue to pulse the mixture. Scrape down the sides of the bowl as needed and pulse until smooth. Taste the pesto and add salt to your liking. I added 1/4 teaspoon. You want the pesto to be slightly saltier than you'd think because it will be spread out thin over the pasta.

3. Cook the pasta according to the package directions (this can done while you make the pesto). Before draining the pasta, reserve about a half cup of the starchy cooking water. Drain the pasta, let cool slightly (about 5 minutes) and then return it to the pot. Add the pesto and stir to coat. If the pasta becomes dry, clumpy, or sticky, use a small amount of the pasta water to help loosen it up. Serve warm!

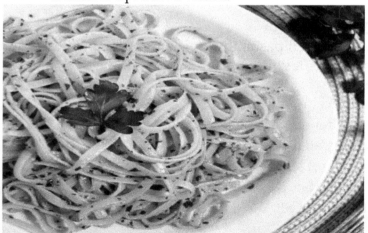

Nutrition Facts: Calories: 361, Carbohydrates: 44g, Fat: 16g, Sodium: 194mg, Protein: 9.49g, Fiber: 2.1g

29. Mediterranean Chickpea Salad

A pretty, colorful vegan Mediterranean chickpea salad for a filling lunch or as a side dish to your grilled meats.

Ingredients:

For the salad:

1. 1 can (15.5 oz) chickpeas, drained and washed
2. 1 cup red onion diced
3. 1 1/3 cup cucumber diced
4. 1 1/2 cup tomato diced
5. 1 medium red bell pepper diced
6. 1/4 cup parsley chopped.

For the dressing:

1. 2 tablespoons olive oil
2. 1/3 cup lemon juice
3. 1 teaspoon ground cumin
4. 1/2 teaspoon ground cardamom
5. 1/2 tablespoon ground dry mint
6. 1 teaspoon Salt or to your liking

Method:

1. In a bowl, combine veggies and set aside.
2. In an empty jar combine salad dressing ingredients and shake well to combine.
3. Pour dressing over veggies and toss to coat everything well.
4. Let it set for 30 minutes in the fridge before serving.

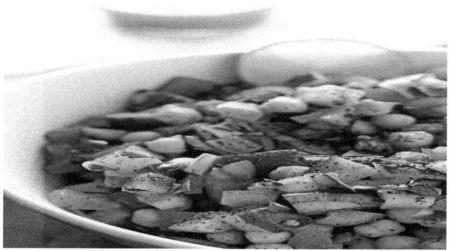

Nutrition Facts: Calories: 131, Carbohydrates: 16.5g, Fat: 6g, Sodium: 127mg, Protein: 4.6g, Fiber: 5g

30. Spaghetti with Corn & Parsley Pesto
Ingredients:
For the pesto:
1. 1/2 cup toasted pine nuts
2. 1/2 cup grated pecorino romano, plus extra to serve
3. 4 cups parsley leaves (tightly packed)
4. 3/4 cup olive oil
5. Salt and pepper, to taste

For the pasta:
1. 1 pound whole wheat spaghetti

2. 1 tablespoon olive oil
3. 2 large shallots, thinly sliced
4. 3 medium garlic cloves, minced
5. 2 cups fresh or frozen corn (from 4 ears of corn; defrost frozen corn before using)

Method:
1. Prepare the pesto in a food processor. Start by pulsing the toasted pine nuts until coarsely ground. Add the pecorino, parsley leaves, and olive oil. Pulse a few times, scrape the bowl with a spatula and pulse a few more times, making sure not to over-blend the pesto. Season to taste with salt and freshly ground black pepper.
2. Bring a large pot of salted water to a boil and cook the pasta until al dente. Meanwhile, heat the olive oil for the pasta in a large pan over a medium heat. Add the sliced shallots to the pan, and cook until softened, about 1 minute. Add the minced garlic and cook for another minute, or until soft and fragrant. Add the corn kernels and a pinch of salt and cook for about 5 minutes, stirring occasionally. Don't overcook the corn — you want some crunch!
3. Strain the spaghetti, then transfer it back to the pot. Add the pesto and toss to coat. Fold in the corn mixture and season to taste with salt and pepper.
4. Serve with extra grated pecorino on top.

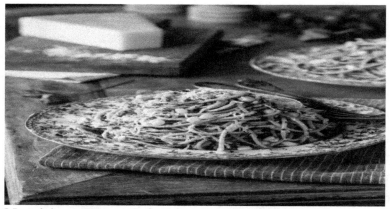

Nutrition Facts: Calories: 614, Carbohydrates: 57g, Fat: 44g, Sodium: 427mg, Protein: 10.4g, Fiber: 9.9g

31. Confit Chicken with Cipollini Onions

What happens when you cook with a lot of oil? Magic. Because oil conducts heat much more efficiently than air, foods that are confited in it, like these chicken thighs, come out incredibly moist and infused with the oil's flavor.

Ingredients:

1. 8 skin-on, bone-in chicken thighs
2. 1 lemon, thinly sliced into rounds, seeds removed
3. 1 teaspoon fennel seeds
4. 6 sprigs rosemary, divided
5. 2 1/2 teaspoon kosher salt, plus more
6. Freshly ground black pepper
7. 1 1/2 pounds baby Yukon Gold potatoes, scrubbed
8. 12 ounces cipollini onions, peeled
9. 4–4 1/2 cups extra-virgin olive oil

Method:

1. Toss chicken thighs, lemon slices, fennel seeds, 4 rosemary sprigs, and 2 1/2 teaspoon salt in a large bowl to combine, then season generously with pepper. Cover and chill at least 12 hours and up to 1 day. Let chicken come to room temperature, 20–25 minutes.
2. Place racks in top and middle of oven; preheat to 275°F. Arrange potatoes and onions in a large Dutch oven or other heavy pot and season with salt. Transfer chicken mixture to pot, scraping in any stray fennel seeds, and arrange chicken thighs, skin side up, over potatoes and onions in a single layer (it will be a tight squeeze).
3. Pour in 4 cups oil. It should come to just over the top of the chicken; if the pieces aren't quite submerged, add the additional 1/2 cup oil. Cover pot and place on middle rack in oven. Bake chicken, adding remaining rosemary sprigs after 1 hour, until meat is very tender but not quite falling off the bone, 2–2 1/2 hours. Let sit until pot is cool enough to handle, 25–30 minutes.
4. Meanwhile, heat broiler. Use tongs to carefully remove chicken from pot and place, skin side up, on a rimmed baking sheet. Transfer potatoes to baking sheet, arranging around chicken. Broil until chicken skin and potatoes are browned and crisp, about 5 minutes. Let rest 5–10 minutes on baking sheet. While chicken and potatoes are under the broiler, transfer onions, lemon slices, and rosemary to a platter.
5. Strain oil through a fine-mesh sieve into a large measuring glass. Use a fork to lightly smash potatoes, revealing some of their creamy interior. Season with more salt. Transfer chicken and potatoes to platter with reserved onions, lemon slices, and rosemary sprigs. Drizzle with some of the strained oil.

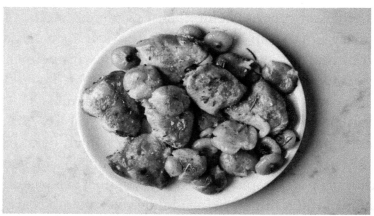

Nutrition Facts: Calories: 510, Carbohydrates: 33g, Fat: 41g, Sodium: 5mg, Protein: 4g, Fiber: 3g

32. Stuffed Onions with Spiced Lamb and Pomegranate
Ingredients:
1. 2 large Spanish onions (1 pound), peeled and left whole
2. 2 tablespoons extra-virgin olive oil, plus more for drizzling
3. 1/4 pound ground lamb
4. 1 1/2 oil-packed anchovies, drained, patted dry, and finely chopped
5. 1/2 tablespoon kosher salt
6. 1/2 teaspoon freshly ground black pepper
7. 3/4 cup raw jasmine rice
8. 1/4 teaspoon ground allspice
9. 1/4 teaspoon ground cinnamon
10. 1 pinch ground nutmeg
11. 3 cups low-sodium chicken broth, divided
12. 3 tablespoons pomegranate molasses, divided
13. 1 tablespoon chopped parsley, plus more for garnish
14. 1 tablespoon chopped cilantro, plus more for garnish
15. 3 tablespoons tomato paste

16. 1/4 cup pomegranate seeds, for garnish

Method:

1. Boil the onions: Fill a medium pot with enough water to cover the onions and bring to a boil. Add whole onions, return to a boil, and cook until tender, 20 to 25 minutes. Using a slotted spoon, remove onions to a colander, drain, and let stand until cool enough to handle. Cut a 1/2-inch wedge from the outside to the core of each onion, then carefully peel 5 outer layers from each onion and reserve; chop the onion wedges and core, and reserve separately.

2. Make the stuffing: In a medium skillet, heat the oil over medium-high. Add the chopped onion and cook, stirring, until golden, 4 to 5 minutes. Add the lamb, anchovies, salt, and pepper and cook, breaking meat up with a wooden spoon, until lamb is no longer pink, 5 to 6 minutes. Add the rice and cook, stirring, until translucent, 2 to 3 minutes. Add the spices and 1 cup broth; cook, stirring, until evaporated, 4 to 5 minutes. Transfer lamb mixture to a rimmed baking sheet and cool slightly; cover and refrigerate for 30 minutes. Remove from the refrigerator, transfer to a bowl, and add parsley, cilantro, and 1 tablespoon pomegranate molasses.

3. Stuff and bake the onions: Preheat the oven to 250°F. In a small bowl, whisk together the remaining broth and pomegranate molasses with the tomato paste. Wrap one onion layer around about 2 to 3 tablespoons filling and arrange seam-side down in a 2-quart shallow baking dish. Repeat with remaining onion layers and filling. Pour liquid over stuffed onions, cover with foil, and roast until tender and some of the liquid is

absorbed, 2 hours (you can roast for up to 3 additional hours for softer, more savory onions). Remove from oven and uncover. Preheat broiler and broil until golden brown, 1 to 2 minutes. Let cool for 10 minutes. To serve, drizzle with oil, and garnish with pomegranate seeds, parsley, and cilantro.

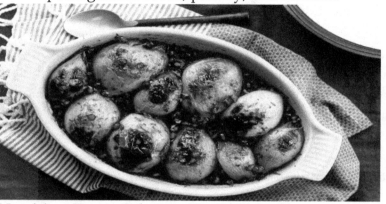

Nutrition Facts: Calories: 99, Carbohydrates: 14.4g, Fat: 3.8g, Sodium: 50.1mg, Protein: 2.3g, Fiber: 2.4g

33. Creamed Pearl Onions and Fennel with Crispy Spiced Breadcrumbs
Ingredients:
1. 4 tablespoons (1/2 stick) unsalted butter, melted, divided
2. 1 large fennel bulb with fronds
3. 2 (12-ounce) bags frozen pearl onions, thawed
4. Kosher salt
5. 1 1/3 cups heavy cream
6. Finely grated zest from 1 orange
7. 1 cup panko (Japanese breadcrumbs) or coarse plain breadcrumbs
8. 1/2 cup finely grated Parmesan
9. 1/3 cup finely chopped flat-leaf parsley

10. 1/4 teaspoon freshly ground black pepper
11. 1/4 teaspoon red pepper flakes

Method:
1. Position rack in middle of oven and preheat to 400°F. Brush a 2-qt. gratin or baking dish, preferably oval or rectangular, with 1/2 Tbsp. butter. Cut fennel bulb and stems into 1/4" pieces.
2. Finely chop 2 tablespoon fennel fronds; set aside. Combine onions, fennel bulb and stems, 1/4 tsp. salt, and 3/4 cup water in a large saucepan. Bring to a boil over high heat, stirring occasionally. Reduce heat to medium, cover, and simmer 5 minutes.
3. Drain onion mixture, pat dry, and transfer to prepared dish. Bring cream and 1/2 tsp. salt to a boil in a small saucepan over medium-high heat, then pour over onion mixture. Bake 15 minutes.
4. Meanwhile, combine orange zest, breadcrumbs, cheese, parsley, black pepper, red pepper flakes, reserved fennel fronds, 1/2 teaspoon salt, and remaining 3 1/2 tablespoon melted butter in a medium bowl.
5. Remove onion mixture from oven and top with breadcrumb mixture. Return to oven and continue baking until breadcrumbs are deep golden brown and cream is bubbling around the edges, 25–30 minutes. Let rest 10 minutes before serving.

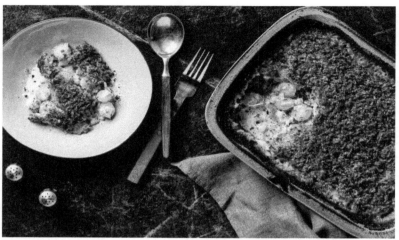

Nutrition Facts: Calories: 112, Carbohydrates: 12.4g, Fat: 6.1g, Sodium: 55mg, Protein: 2.5g, Fiber: 1.2g

34. Roasted strawberry and cream pie

This pie plays on the classic combination of strawberries and cream that you grew up on as a child. This adult version is perfect for relaxed weekend entertaining.

Ingredients:

1. 435g frozen Careme vanilla bean pastry, thawed, or other store-bought sweet short crust rolled to a thickness of 3mm
2. 750g strawberries, hulled, halved if large
3. 1 vanilla bean, split, seeds scraped
4. 2 tablespoon maple syrup
5. 1 thyme sprig, plus extra to decorate
6. 500g mascarpone cheese
7. 11/2 cups (375ml) thickened cream
8. 1/3 cup (40g) pure icing sugar
9. 1 teaspoon vanilla bean paste

Method:

1. Preheat oven to 200°C. Line base and side of a 22cm × 5cm-deep pie dish with pastry and trim away the excess. Line pastry case with baking paper and fill with baking beads (or uncooked rice or dried beans).

2. Place on a baking tray. Cook for 20 minutes or until golden, then remove baking beads and paper. Cook for a further 5 minutes or until base is dry to the touch. Set aside and leave to cool completely. Keep oven on.

3. Toss together strawberries, vanilla pod and seeds, maple syrup and thyme on a baking tray lined with baking paper, and roast for 16 minutes or until softened and slightly syrupy. Cool to room temperature. 4. Whisk mascarpone, cream, icing sugar and vanilla bean paste in a bowl until thick.

4. How to whip cream 5. Spread into the cooled pie crust and top with roasted strawberries and their syrup.

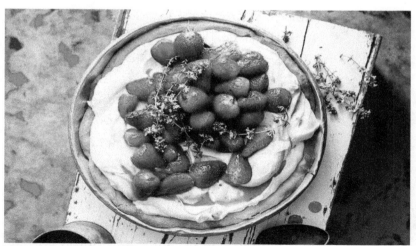

Nutrition Facts: Calories: 125, Carbohydrates: 18.4g, Fat: 3.5g, Sodium: 200mg, Protein: 3g, Fiber: 0.9g

35. Carrot pizza with fontina and red onion

Ingredients:
1. 1/4 cup mascarpone
2. 1/8 teaspoon cayenne pepper

For the pizza:
1. 1/2 pound prepared pizza dough, room temperature
2. All-purpose flour (for surface)
3. Olive oil (for brushing)
4. 8 ounces Fontina cheese, grated (about 2 cups)
5. 1/2 medium red onion, root intact and thinly sliced lengthwise into wedges
6. 1 cup (loosely packed) carrot fronds or baby arugula

Method:
1. For the carrot puree: Heat oil in a large skillet over medium-high until shimmering. Add onions and cook, stirring often, until translucent, about 2 minutes. Add carrots and cook, stirring occasionally, until beginning to brown, about 5 minutes, then add wine and cook, stirring often, until reduced by half, about 2 minutes.
2. Reduce heat to medium-low, add salt and 1 cup water, and stir to combine. Cover and simmer until carrots are tender and most of the liquid has evaporated, about 15 minutes. Transfer mixture to a blender. Add mascarpone, cayenne, and 1/4 cup water. Remove stopper from lid or leave lid slightly ajar, cover with a towel (hot liquids can splatter), and purée until smooth.
3. For the pizza: Place 2 overturned rimmed baking sheets in the upper and lower thirds of oven and preheat to 450°F. Divide dough in half on a lightly floured surface and form into 2 balls. Roll out balls into ovals about 6x10 inches in size (make sure they fit on baking sheets).

4. Remove preheated sheets from oven and brush bottoms with oil. Carefully place dough on sheets and brush with more oil. Return to oven and bake until dough is beginning to brown, about 5 minutes. Spread reserved carrot purée evenly on pizzas, then sprinkle with cheese and onion. Return to oven and bake pizzas, rotating the sheets and swapping their positions on the oven racks halfway through, until cheese is melted and bubbling, 10–12 minutes. Transfer pizzas to cutting boards, top with carrot fronds, and slice.

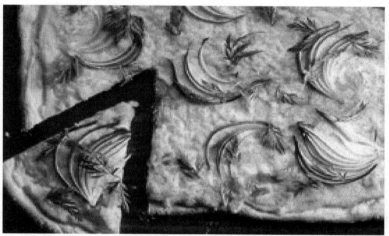

Nutrition Facts: Calories: 103, Carbohydrates: 19.9g, Fat: 0.4g, Sodium: 29.3mg, Protein: 3.6g, Fiber: 2.8g

36. Chickpea Salad with Red Onion, Sumac, and Lemon

Ingredients:
1. 3 cups uncooked chickpeas
2. 4 cloves garlic, smashed
3. Salt and freshly ground black pepper
4. 1 large red onion, sliced very thin
5. 1 tablespoon sumac
6. 1 teaspoon chili powder
7. 1 teaspoon salt
8. 1 bunch Italian parsley, leaves finely chopped
9. 1 large lemon, juiced (about 3 tablespoons)
10. 2 tablespoons extra-virgin olive oil
11. 2 tablespoons pomegranate syrup
12. 5 to 6 sprigs fresh mint

Method:
1. Cover the chickpeas with water in a large bowl and soak overnight. Or do a fast soak: Cover with an inch of water in a saucepan and bring to a boil. Turn off the heat, cover, and soak for 1 hour.
2. Drain the soaked chickpeas. Cover with fresh water and stir in the garlic cloves and a few pinches of salt and pepper. Bring to a boil then lower the heat and simmer for 60 minutes to 2 hours, or until just tender but not falling apart. You can also cook them in the pressure cooker for about 40 minutes (or according to your pressure cooker instructions). When cooked, spread on a large baking sheet to cool.
3. While the chickpeas are cooling, peel and quarter the onion. Shave it as thin as possible into a large bowl, using a very sharp knife or a mandoline. Stir in the sumac, chili powder, and salt. Use your hands to

massage the spices and salt into the onions for several minutes. Drain off any liquid that develops in the bottom of the bowl.

4. Add the chickpeas and chopped parsley to the onions and use your hands or two forks to toss everything thoroughly. Whisk together the lemon juice, olive oil, and pomegranate syrup and toss with the salad. Season to taste with salt and pepper. Continue tossing until the onions are fully incorporated and no longer in small clumps. Refrigerate until serving (this salad gets better overnight).

5. Just before serving, finely chop the mint leaves and sprinkle over the salad.

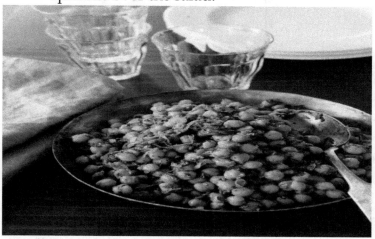

Nutrition Facts: Calories: 40, Carbohydrates: 5g, Fat: 2g, Sodium: 110mg, Protein: 1g, Fiber: 2g

37. Red-Wine Risotto

Ingredients:

1. 4 1/2 cups reduced-sodium beef broth
2. 2 tablespoon extra-virgin olive oil
3. 1 medium onion, finely chopped
4. 2 cloves garlic, minced
5. 1 1/2 cups risotto rice
6. 1/4 teaspoon salt
7. 1 3/4 cups dry red wine
8. 2 teaspoons tomato paste
9. 1 cup finely shredded Parmigiano-Reggiano cheese, divided
10. Freshly ground pepper, to taste

Method:

1. Place broth in a medium saucepan; bring to a simmer over medium-high heat. Reduce the heat so the broth remains steaming, but is not simmering.
2. Heat oil in a Dutch oven over medium-low heat. Add onion and cook, stirring occasionally, for 5 minutes. Add garlic and cook, stirring, until the onion is very soft and translucent, about 2 minutes. Add rice and salt and stir to coat.
3. Stir 1/2 cup of the hot broth and a generous splash of wine into the rice; reduce heat to a gentle simmer and cook, stirring constantly, until the liquid has been absorbed. Add more broth, 1/2 cup at a time along with some wine, stirring after each addition until most of the liquid has been absorbed.
4. After about 10 minutes, stir in tomato paste. Continue to cook, adding broth and wine and stirring after each addition until most of the liquid is absorbed; the risotto is done when you've used all the broth and wine and

the rice is creamy and just tender, 20 to 30 minutes more.

5. Remove the risotto from the heat; stir in 3/4 cup cheese and pepper. Serve sprinkled with the remaining 1/4 cup cheese.

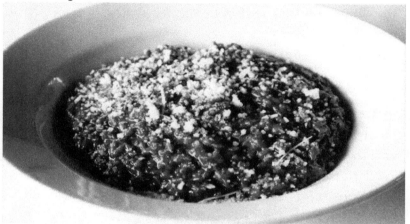

Nutrition Facts: Calories: 253, Carbohydrates: 31g, Fat: 4g, Sodium: 493mg, Protein: 7g, Fiber: 1g

38. Beans in red wine

A great vegetarian dish with a deep, savory flavor

Ingredients:

1. 2 red onions, finely diced
2. 2 garlic cloves, crushed
3. 2 celery sticks, chopped

4. 115g red lentils
5. 1 tablespoon chopped fresh thyme
6. 300ml red wine
7. 1 x 400g tin chopped tomatoes
8. 1 x 400g tin kidney beans in water, drained and rinsed
9. 1 x 400g tin cannellini beans in water, drained and rinsed
10. 2 teaspoon vegetable stock powder
11. black pepper

Method:

1. Heat a large, non-stick pan, add the onions and garlic and dry fry until soft.
2. Add the celery, lentils and thyme. Pour in the wine, tomatoes and kidney beans, then stir in the stock powder.
3. Bring to the boil, then reduce to a gentle simmer. Simmer for 20 minutes, until the lentils are soft, adding a little water if required. Season to taste.

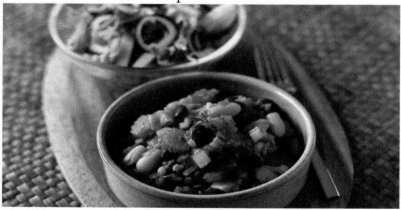

Nutrition Facts: Calories: 60, Carbohydrates: 23g, Fat: 0g, Sodium: 0mg, Protein: 9g, Fiber: 16g

39. Ramp fritters
Ingredients:
1. 1 cup all-purpose flour
2. 3/4 cup rice flour
3. 1 teaspoon baking powder
4. 1 teaspoon sugar
5. 1 teaspoon kosher salt
6. 3/4 cup club soda
7. 3/4 cup light beer
8. 10 oz. ramps, trimmed, cut into 1" pieces
9. Vegetable oil (for frying; about 6 cups)
10. Lemon wedges, for serving

Method:
1. Remove any slippery outer layers from ramp bulbs, trim roots, then soak in a bowl of cold water, swishing around gently to loosen any dirt. Lift out ramps and blot dry with paper towels. Avoid cramming them in a salad spinner so as not to damage the delicate leaves. Cut ramps into 1" pieces (you should get about 5 cups).
2. Whisk all-purpose flour, rice flour, baking powder, sugar, and salt in a large bowl to combine. Make a well in the center and pour in club soda and beer; whisk until smooth.
3. Fold in ramps. Pour oil into a large cast-iron skillet fitted with thermometer to come 1" up sides and heat over medium-high until thermometer registers 350°F. Working in batches, place 1/4-cup mounds of batter into skillet and press down lightly to flatten and submerge.
4. Fry, turning once, until fritters are golden brown, about 4 minutes. Transfer to paper towels to drain; sprinkle with salt. Serve with lemon wedges for squeezing over.

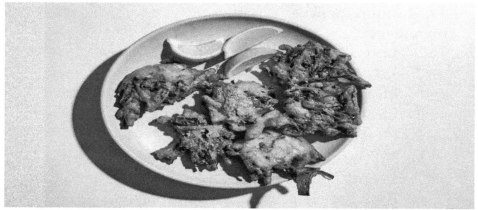

Nutrition Facts: Calories: 146, Carbohydrates: 15.3g, Fat: 6.4g, Sodium: 128mg, Protein: 4.7g, Fiber: 1.1g

40. Cheesecake with strawberry crumble

Ingredients:

1. 2 teaspoon ground ginger
2. 400g shortbread biscuits, chopped
3. 140g unsalted butter, melted
4. 250g white chocolate, chopped
5. 3 titanium-strength gelatine leaves
6. 750g cream cheese, softened
7. 1 cup (220g) caster sugar
8. 150ml thickened cream
9. 250ml creme fraiche
10. Black sesame seeds and freeze-dried strawberries, to serve

Method:

1. Grease a 23cm spring form cake pan and line the base and sides with baking paper.
2. Place ginger and 250g biscuit in a food processor and whiz to fine crumbs. Add 80g butter and pulse to combine. Press into base of prepared pan, then chill for 30 minutes to firm up.

3. Place chocolate in a heatproof bowl set over a pan of simmering water (don't let the bowl touch the water) and stir until melted and smooth.
4. Soak the gelatine in a bowl of cold water for 5 minutes to soften. Meanwhile, whiz the cream cheese and sugar in a food processor until smooth.
5. Squeeze any excess water from the gelatine, then place in a bowl with 2 tablespoon hot water, stirring to dissolve. Add to food processor with the chocolate, cream and creme fraiche, and whiz until smooth. Pour over base and chill for 4 hours or until set.
6. Preheat oven to 180°C. To make the crumble, place remaining 60g butter and 150g biscuit in a food processor and whiz until just crushed. Spread over a baking tray and bake, stirring once, for 12 minutes, or until golden. Cool completely.
7. To serve, remove cake from pan. Scatter over the crumb, then top with sesame and freeze-dried strawberries.

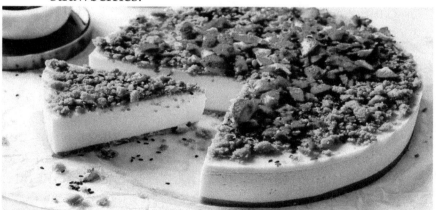

Nutrition Facts: Calories: 175, Carbohydrates: 24g, Fat: 7.8g, Sodium: 0mg, Protein: 2.3g, Fiber: 1g

41. Strawberry- Graham Galette

Ingredients:

1. graham crackers (about 3.7 ounces)
2. ¾ teaspoon kosher salt
3. ⅔ cup all-purpose flour, plus more for rolling
4. 5 tablespoons sugar, divided
5. 2 large eggs
6. ½ cup (1 stick) unsalted butter, melted, cooled, divided
7. 1 pound strawberries, hulled, sliced
8. 1 lime (½ teaspoon finely grated zest and 1 teaspoon fresh juice)
9. ½ cup very cold heavy cream

Method:

1. Place a rack in bottom third of oven; preheat to 350°. Place graham crackers in a large resealable plastic bag and zip it up, pressing out most of the air. Using a wine bottle or rolling pin, firmly roll over crackers several times, crushing them into fine crumbs (some larger crumbs are okay).
2. Measure out 1 cup crumbs (which should be almost all of them) and transfer to a medium bowl. Add salt, ⅔ cup flour, and 2 tablespoon sugar. Mix with a fork to combine, then add 1 egg and 6 tablespoon melted butter.
3. Mix with fork until dough forms, then knead with your hands inside of bowl until no floury spots remain and dough is smooth. It'll be a little soft and slightly oily, which is fine!
4. Lightly flour a piece of parchment paper and place dough on top. Lightly flour top of dough, then cover with another piece of parchment.

5. Using bottle or rolling pin, roll dough into a round (it doesn't have to be perfect!) about 12" in diameter and ⅛" thick. Periodically peel back parchment and dust with more flour to prevent sticking. Slide entire sheet of parchment paper onto a rimmed baking sheet.

6. Sprinkle 1 tablespoon sugar over surface of dough, leaving about a 2" border. Pile strawberries into center of dough and arrange in an even layer, leaving the same 2" border.

7. Sprinkle strawberries with 1 tablespoon sugar and drizzle with remaining 2 tablespoon butter.

8. Using a micro plane or fine grater, grate zest of about one-half of lime over strawberries. Cut off half of lime with no zest and squeeze juice over strawberries. Save the other half for later. Using edges of parchment to help lift, fold empty border of dough up and over strawberries, working your way around in roughly 2" sections, overlapping folds as needed. Press all the way around to secure folds and keep dough in place. It might crack or tear in places, but don't worry! Just pinch it back together.

9. Brush top of border with remaining egg wash and sprinkle with remaining 1 tablespoon sugar. Bake Galette until crust is browned around the edges and juices from strawberries are syrupy and actively bubbling, 40–45 minutes. If some juices escape and end up on the parchment paper, don't worry — the parchment will prevent the tart from sticking. Let cool at least 20 minutes.

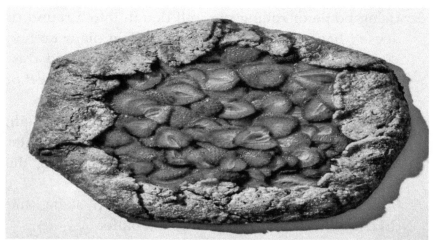

Nutrition Facts: Calories: 20, Carbohydrates: 4.5g, Fat: 0.1g, Sodium: 0.3mg, Protein: 0.2g, Fiber: 0.6g

CPSIA information can be obtained
at www.ICGtesting.com
Printed in the USA
BVHW050544120421
604724BV00002B/347